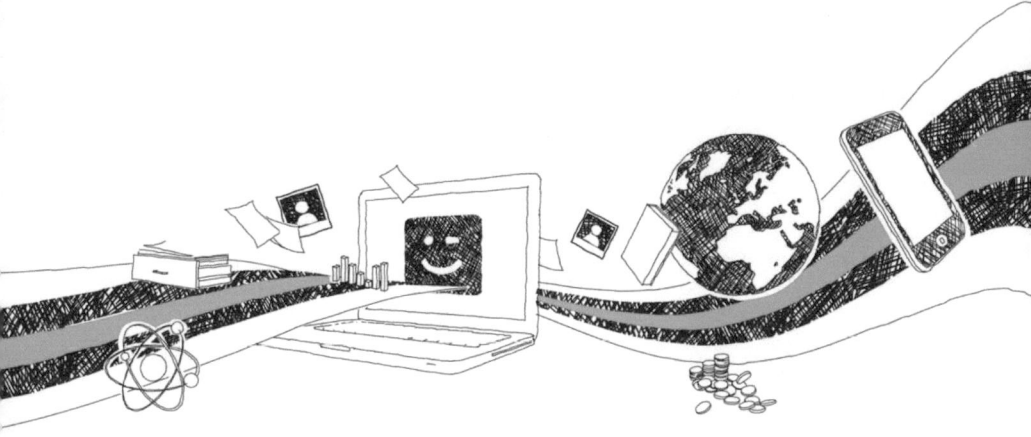
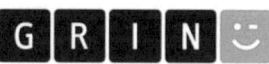

Carol Benjamin

H1N1 Virus and Mortality in Blacks and Hispanic Children with Asthma

GRIN Publishing

Bibliographic information published by the German National Library:

The German National Library lists this publication in the National Bibliography; detailed bibliographic data are available on the Internet at http://dnb.dnb.de .

Imprint:

Copyright © 2010 GRIN Verlag GmbH
Print and binding: Books on Demand GmbH, Norderstedt Germany
ISBN: 978-3-656-55123-2

This book at GRIN:

http://www.grin.com/en/e-book/265476/h1n1-virus-and-mortality-in-blacks-and-hispanic-children-with-asthma

GRIN - Your knowledge has value

Since its foundation in 1998, GRIN has specialized in publishing academic texts by students, college teachers and other academics as e-book and printed book. The website www.grin.com is an ideal platform for presenting term papers, final papers, scientific essays, dissertations and specialist books.

Visit us on the internet:

http://www.grin.com/

http://www.facebook.com/grincom

http://www.twitter.com/grin_com

H1N1 Virus and Mortality in

Black and Hispanic Children with Asthma

Carol Benjamin

TUI University

Abstract

This Session Long Project Part 1 - involves a critical analysis of a H1N1 Virus and

Mortality in Black and Hispanic Children with Asthma. The topic is focused on the

relationship between these two theoretical variables. The topic was introduced by clearly

identifying the two variables. Previous research was cited and the hypothesized

associations between the two variables as well as the direction of that relationship were

discussed. The historical development of the theory connecting the two variables was

discussed.

Part I - Introduce your topic by clearly identifying the two variables that are of interest to you. Citing previous research, state the hypothesized association between the two variables as well as the direction(s) of that relationship. Briefly trace the historical development of the theory connecting the two variables.

Topic: H1NI virus and Mortality among Black and Hispanic Children with Asthma.

The H1N1 virus is a variable that is of interest and will be discussed as one of the variables in the study. A new research by an anonymous author from the University of California reveals recent research from the United States, which shows that, in the year 1977, H1N1 influenza A virus reappeared after a 20-year absence. Genetic analysis indicated that this strain was missing decades of nucleotide sequence evolution, suggesting an accidental release of a frozen laboratory strain into the general population.

The author shows that recently, this strain and its descendants were included in an analysis attempting to date the origin of pandemic influenza virus without accounting for the missing decades of evolution. Here, we investigated the effect of using viral isolates with biologically unrealistic sampling dates on estimates of divergence dates. Not accounting for missing sequence evolution produced biased results and increased the variance of date estimates of the most recent common ancestor of the re-emergent lineages and across the entire phylogeny. Reanalysis of the H1N1 sequences excluding isolates with unrealistic sampling dates indicates that the 1977 re-emergent lineage was circulating for approximately one year before detection, making it difficult to determine the geographic source of reintroduction.

Mortality in Black and Hispanic children with asthma is another variable that will be discussed. An article by Ayi (2006) shows black children are 25 percent more likely to die and 50 percent more likely to be hospitalized for asthma, according to a report in the February issue of the Journal of Allergy and Clinical Immunology. The author also explains that asthma-related death rates have remained about the same for white children as well as hospitalization rates have decreased. However hospitalization and death rates for Black children have increased. The research conducted by Ayi (2006) showed that nationally, an average of 12 white children died from asthma each year, but an average of 46 Black died from the same condition.

Previous studies have hypothesized association between H1N1 virus and mortality in African American children with asthma. Article from Center for Disease Control and Prevention shows from April 2009 to September 2009, almost one-third of people hospitalized with complications from 2009 H1N1 influenza were persons with asthma. Asthma-related hospitalization and mortality rates from all causes, not just influenza, are approximately two to three times higher among non-Hispanic blacks compared with non-Hispanic whites.

Austin (2009) article states that the Center for Disease Control report also shows that Black and Hispanic children have suffered higher proportional death rates from the H1N1 virus than their white counterparts. The author also argued that Blacks and Hispanics are represented in a greater proportion among seasonal and H1N1 deaths in children than their representation in the United States population. The reasons for more severe outcomes among Black and Hispanics are unknown but may be related to the frequency of underlying conditions that increase the risk for influenza complications in that population or the timing of medical care and or treatment.

A review of the literature shows that an increase in poverty which is dominant among African American increases the mortality rate from H1N1 virus. Austin mentioned Dr. Louis Sullivan the former president and founder of the Morehouse School of Medicine who agrees with the arguments of Center for Disease Control. Sullivan states that African Americans and Hispanics have a high concentration in low-income neighborhoods. Poor communities have higher incidents of asthma. This is one condition that increases susceptibility to influenza. Sullivan also states that the lack of well-balanced meals and accurate nutritional awareness plays a role in the deaths.

The H1N1 pandemic started in the 2009 spring. From the literature reviewed from 2009 to present, the H1N1 virus causes increased mortality among Black and Hispanic children with Asthma. Article written by Hennessy- Fiske (2010) reports that California Latinos have been nearly twice as likely as whites to die of H1N1 flu since the pandemic began last spring, according to statewide figures released by the California Department of Public Health.

Over the same months, blacks in the state have been 50% more likely to die of H1N1 flu than whites, the report said. Chavez an epidemiologist who contributed to this article states that blacks were three times as likely as whites to be hospitalized with H1N1 flu, and Latinos twice as likely. Native Americans, who make up most of the "other" category in state H1N1 data, are also more likely to be hospitalized and die of H1N1 flu than whites. The new statewide figures came out less than a week after Los Angeles County health officials released data showing H1N1, also known as swine flu, had disproportionately struck the young and minorities in the county.

Reference

Anonymous, (2010). H1N1 Virus; Research from University of California, Department
of Pathology in h1n1virus provides new insights. Obesity, Fitness & Wellness
Week. Retrieved on July 18, 2010 from:
http://proquest.umi.com/pqdweb?index=1&did=2074281841&SrchMode=1&sid=
1&Fmt=3&VInst=PROD&VType=PQD&RQT=309&VName=PQD&TS=12794
85087&clientId=29440
Article from Center for Disease Control on line.

Austin, N. (2009). H1N1 deaths of Black, Hispanic children higher than for whites
Chicago Defender. Retrieved on July 18, 2010 from:
http://proquest.umi.com/pqdweb?index=0&did=1929145481&SrchMode=1&sid=
1&Fmt=6&VInst=PROD&VType=PQD&RQT=309&VName=PQD&TS=12795
08297&clientId=29440

Ayi, M. (2006). Asthma deaths and hospitalization more likely for Black kids.
Chicago Defender. Vol. XCIX, iss.421; pg 3 Retrieved on July 18, 2010 from:
http://proquest.umi.com/pqdweb?index=43&did=1016889031&SrchMode=1&sid
=6&Fmt=3&VInst=PROD&VType=PQD&RQT=309&VName=PQD&TS=1279
505897&clientId=29440

Center for Disease Control

Hennessy-Fiske, M. (2010). H1N1 death rates higher for some ethnic; groups; blacks

and Native Americans in the state have been more likely to die than whites.

Los Angeles Times. Retrieved on July 19, 2010 from:

http://proquest.umi.com/pqdweb?index=2&did=1939710191&SrchMode=1&sid=

8&Fmt=3&VInst=PROD&VType=PQD&RQT=309&VName=PQD&TS=12795

95778&clientId=29440

.